STAGE 4 RENAL DIET COOKBOOK FOR SENIORS

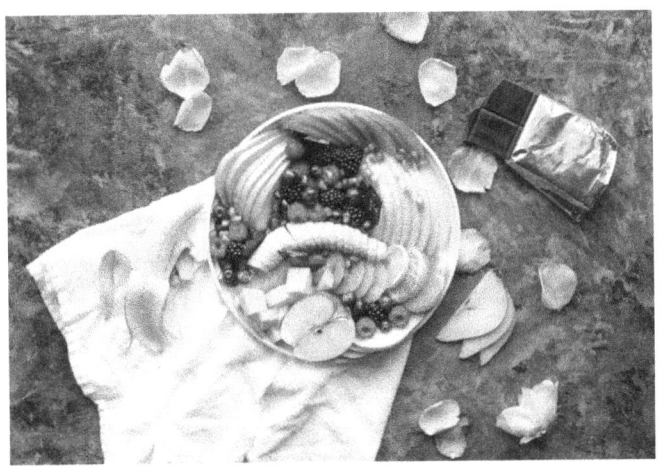

DR. JESSICA SMITH

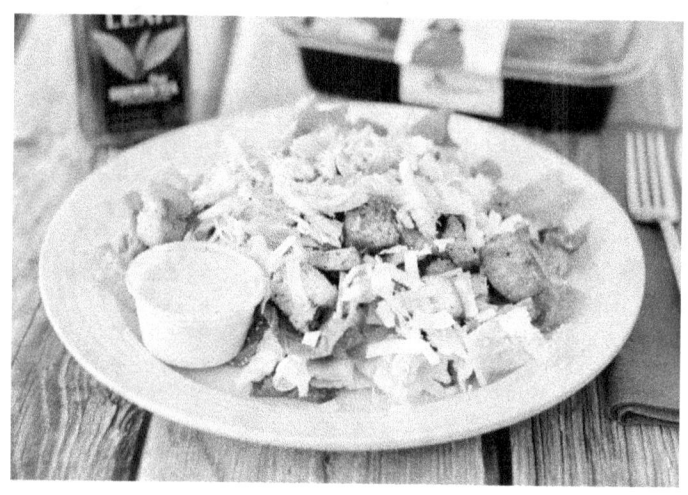

TABLE OF CONTENTS

CHAPTER ONE

How to Use this Cookbook

Understand Dietary Restrictions: Research and understand the dietary restrictions for individuals in Stage 4 renal disease. Key considerations typically include limiting phosphorus, potassium, sodium, and protein intake while ensuring adequate nutrition.

Consult with a Dietitian: Work closely with a registered dietitian specializing in renal nutrition to ensure the recipes meet the specific dietary needs of seniors in Stage 4 kidney disease.

Develop Recipe Guidelines: Establish guidelines for recipe development, emphasizing low phosphorus, low potassium, low sodium, and moderate protein content. Incorporate senior-friendly cooking methods and ingredients.

Focus on Nutrient Balance: Design recipes that emphasize nutrient balance and variety. Include a variety of fruits, vegetables, lean proteins, and whole grains while avoiding high-phosphorus and high-potassium ingredients.

Create Simple Recipes: Keep recipes simple and easy to follow, considering the physical limitations that some seniors may have. Use clear instructions and minimize the number of ingredients required.

Provide Portion Control Information: Offer portion control information with each recipe to help seniors manage their intake of key nutrients. This can include serving sizes and nutritional breakdowns per serving.

Offer Substitution Suggestions: Provide substitution suggestions for ingredients that may need to be limited due to renal restrictions. For example, suggest lower potassium alternatives for high-potassium ingredients.

Incorporate Flavorful Herbs and Spices: Enhance the flavor of dishes without relying on salt by incorporating a variety of herbs, spices, and other flavorings. Experiment with different combinations to keep meals interesting.

Include Tips for Meal Planning: Offer meal planning tips and suggestions to help seniors maintain a balanced renal diet throughout the week. This can include batch cooking, meal prepping, and storage recommendations.

Provide Educational Resources: Supplement the cookbook with educational resources on renal nutrition, including information on reading food labels, managing fluid intake, and making healthy food choices outside of the home.

Understanding Stage 4 Renal Diet for Seniors

Understanding the Stage 4 renal diet is crucial for seniors managing advanced kidney disease.

At this stage, the kidneys have significantly reduced function, making it essential to carefully control nutrient intake to prevent further damage and manage symptoms effectively.

The primary goals of the Stage 4 renal diet for seniors are to reduce the workload on the kidneys and manage complications associated with impaired kidney function.

This often involves restrictions on certain nutrients, including phosphorus, potassium, sodium, and protein.

Phosphorus restriction is essential because impaired kidneys struggle to excrete excess phosphorus, leading to mineral imbalances and bone health issues.

Potassium restriction helps prevent dangerous levels of potassium in the blood, which can affect heart rhythm and muscle function.

Sodium control is important for managing blood pressure and fluid retention. Moderating protein intake reduces the buildup of waste products in the blood, easing the burden on the kidneys.

Seniors in Stage 4 renal disease should focus on consuming a balanced diet that includes controlled amounts of high-quality proteins, limited fruits and vegetables with lower potassium content, and foods with reduced phosphorus and sodium levels.

Working closely with a registered dietitian specializing in renal nutrition is crucial to tailor the diet to individual needs and ensure adequate nutrition while managing kidney disease effectively.

Principles of Stage 4 Renal Diet for Seniors

The principles of the Stage 4 renal diet for seniors revolve around managing the progression of kidney disease and addressing associated complications through careful control of nutrient intake:

Phosphorus Control: Seniors with Stage 4 renal disease need to limit phosphorus intake because impaired kidneys struggle to remove excess phosphorus from the blood. High phosphorus levels can lead to bone and cardiovascular issues. The diet emphasizes choosing foods with lower phosphorus content, such as white bread, rice, and pasta instead of whole grain varieties, and limiting dairy and protein-rich foods.

Potassium Moderation: Potassium levels must be carefully managed as elevated levels can disrupt heart rhythm and muscle function. Seniors are advised to limit high-potassium foods like bananas, oranges, tomatoes, and potatoes, opting for lower-potassium alternatives such as apples, berries, and green beans.

Sodium Restriction: Sodium control is crucial for managing blood pressure and fluid balance. Seniors are encouraged to reduce their sodium intake by avoiding processed foods, canned soups, and salty snacks, while opting for fresh, whole foods and using herbs and spices for flavoring.

Protein Management: Moderating protein intake helps lessen the workload on the kidneys by reducing the buildup of waste products in the blood. Seniors should focus on consuming high-quality proteins in controlled portions, such as lean meats, fish, poultry, eggs, and limited dairy products.

Fluid Management: Seniors may also need to monitor their fluid intake to prevent fluid overload, which can strain the kidneys and lead to complications like edema and high blood pressure. Guidance from a registered dietitian helps seniors strike the right balance between staying hydrated and avoiding excessive fluid intake.

Regular monitoring and adjustments under the guidance of healthcare professionals are essential for personalized management of the renal diet.

Benefits of Stage 4 Renal Diet for Seniors

The Stage 4 renal diet offers numerous benefits for seniors with advanced kidney disease, enhancing their overall health and quality of life:

Slows Disease Progression: Adhering to the renal diet can help slow the progression of kidney disease by reducing the workload on the kidneys and minimizing further damage caused by excessive accumulation of waste products and electrolyte imbalances.

Manages Symptoms: Following the renal diet helps manage common symptoms associated with Stage 4 kidney disease, such as fluid retention, high blood pressure, and bone disorders. By controlling intake of nutrients like sodium, potassium, and phosphorus, seniors can alleviate these symptoms and improve their comfort.

Reduces Complications: By controlling key nutrients, particularly phosphorus and potassium, the renal diet helps reduce the risk of complications such as cardiovascular disease, bone disease, and electrolyte imbalances, which are common in advanced kidney disease.

Improves Nutritional Status: Despite dietary restrictions, the renal diet focuses on providing balanced nutrition tailored to the individual's needs, ensuring adequate intake of essential nutrients like protein, vitamins, and minerals.

Enhances Quality of Life: By promoting better symptom management, slowing disease progression, and supporting overall health, the renal diet ultimately enhances the quality of life for seniors with Stage 4 kidney disease.

It allows them to maintain independence, engage in daily activities with greater ease, and enjoy a more fulfilling lifestyle.

Overall, the Stage 4 renal diet offers seniors with advanced kidney disease a proactive approach to managing their health and well-being, empowering them to live life to the fullest despite their medical condition.

Tips for Stage 4 Renal Diet for Seniors

Managing a Stage 4 renal diet can be challenging for seniors, but with the right strategies, it's possible to maintain health and well-being.

Here are some helpful tips tailored specifically for seniors navigating Stage 4 kidney disease:

Work with a Dietitian: Seek guidance from a registered dietitian specializing in renal nutrition. They can provide personalized recommendations and help create a meal plan that meets individual needs while adhering to renal diet restrictions.

Read Food Labels: Seniors should become familiar with reading food labels to identify hidden sources of phosphorus, potassium, and sodium. Look for keywords like phosphates, potassium chloride, and sodium bicarbonate on packaged foods.

Portion Control: Practice portion control to avoid overloading the body with nutrients that the kidneys may struggle to process. Use measuring cups or visual cues to gauge appropriate serving sizes.

Plan Meals Ahead: Plan meals and snacks in advance to ensure they align with renal diet guidelines. This can help prevent impulsive food choices and ensure a balanced intake throughout the day.

Choose Low-Phosphorus Foods: Opt for foods lower in phosphorus, such as white bread, rice, pasta, and certain fruits and vegetables. Limit high-phosphorus foods like dairy products, nuts, seeds, and whole grains.

Limit High-Potassium Foods: Limit intake of high-potassium foods like bananas, oranges, tomatoes, and potatoes. Instead, choose lower-potassium alternatives such as apples, berries, and green beans.

Cooking Methods: Use cooking methods that reduce the need for added salt, such as grilling, steaming, baking, or roasting. Experiment with herbs, spices, and lemon juice to enhance flavor without increasing sodium intake.

Stay Hydrated: Drink water throughout the day to stay hydrated, but monitor fluid intake closely if advised by a healthcare professional to restrict fluids.

Stay Informed: Stay informed about updates and advancements in renal nutrition. Attend educational sessions or support groups to learn from experts and peers.

Seek Support: Don't hesitate to seek support from family, friends, or support groups. Having a support network can make it easier to navigate dietary changes and stay motivated.

It's essential to approach dietary changes with patience, persistence, and a positive attitude.

Guidelines for Stage 4 Renal Diet for Seniors

Guidelines for a Stage 4 renal diet for seniors are essential for managing kidney disease while maintaining overall health. Here are key principles to consider:

Phosphorus Control: Seniors should limit phosphorus intake to prevent complications like bone disease and cardiovascular issues. Choose low-phosphorus foods such as white bread, rice, pasta, and lean meats, and avoid high-phosphorus items like dairy, nuts, seeds, and whole grains.

Potassium Moderation: Manage potassium levels to prevent heart rhythm disturbances and muscle weakness. Opt for lower-potassium fruits and vegetables like apples, berries, and green beans, and limit high-potassium foods such as bananas, oranges, tomatoes, and potatoes.

Sodium Restriction: Control sodium intake to manage blood pressure and fluid balance. Avoid processed foods, canned soups, and salty snacks, and use herbs, spices, and lemon juice for flavor instead of salt.

Protein Management: Moderation of protein intake helps reduce the burden on the kidneys. Choose high-quality protein sources like lean meats, fish, poultry, eggs, and limited dairy products, and control portion sizes.

Fluid Monitoring: Seniors may need to monitor fluid intake to prevent fluid overload. Follow individualized recommendations from healthcare providers, balancing hydration needs with fluid restrictions.

Regular Monitoring: Regularly monitor kidney function, blood pressure, and other relevant markers with healthcare providers to adjust dietary guidelines as needed.

Collaboration with Healthcare Team: Work closely with a registered dietitian and healthcare team to tailor dietary recommendations to individual needs, considering factors like comorbidities, medications, and lifestyle preferences.

Regular communication with healthcare providers ensures a personalized approach to dietary management of kidney disease.

Causes of Stage 4 Renal Disease

Stage 4 renal disease, also known as Stage 4 chronic kidney disease (CKD), is characterized by severely reduced kidney function, with a glomerular filtration rate (GFR) of 15-29 mL/min/1.73m².

Several factors contribute to the development and progression of Stage 4 renal disease:

Diabetes Mellitus: Diabetes is the leading cause of CKD worldwide.

Prolonged high blood sugar levels can damage the small blood vessels in the kidneys, leading to diabetic nephropathy and CKD progression.

Hypertension (High Blood Pressure): Uncontrolled hypertension can damage the blood vessels in the kidneys, impairing their ability to filter waste products from the blood effectively.

Glomerulonephritis: Glomerulonephritis refers to inflammation of the glomeruli, the tiny filtering units within the kidneys. Chronic inflammation can lead to scarring and permanent damage to the kidneys.

Polycystic Kidney Disease (PKD): PKD is a genetic disorder characterized by the growth of numerous fluid-filled cysts in the kidneys. Over time, these cysts can enlarge and impair kidney function.

Autoimmune Diseases: Conditions like lupus and vasculitis can cause inflammation and damage to the kidneys, leading to CKD.

Obstructive Diseases: Conditions such as kidney stones, tumors, or enlarged prostate glands can obstruct the flow of urine, leading to kidney damage over time.

Recurrent Infections: Chronic or recurrent urinary tract infections can cause scarring and damage to the kidneys, contributing to CKD development.

Medications and Toxins: Certain medications, toxins, and environmental exposures can damage kidney tissue and impair kidney function, leading to CKD progression.

Types of Stage 4 Renal Disease

Stage 4 renal disease, or Stage 4 chronic kidney disease (CKD), encompasses various types of kidney conditions that lead to significant impairment in kidney function.

Some common types of Stage 4 renal disease include:

Diabetic Nephropathy: This type of kidney disease occurs as a complication of diabetes mellitus. Prolonged high blood sugar levels damage the small blood vessels in the kidneys, leading to kidney dysfunction and eventual kidney failure.

Hypertensive Nephropathy: Uncontrolled high blood pressure over time can cause damage to the blood vessels in the kidneys, impairing their ability to filter waste products from the blood effectively.

Glomerulonephritis: Glomerulonephritis refers to inflammation of the glomeruli, the filtering units within the kidneys. Chronic inflammation can lead to scarring and progressive loss of kidney function.

Polycystic Kidney Disease (PKD): PKD is a genetic disorder characterized by the growth of numerous fluid-filled cysts in the kidneys. These cysts can gradually enlarge and replace healthy kidney tissue, leading to kidney failure.

Interstitial Nephritis: Interstitial nephritis involves inflammation of the kidney tubules and surrounding tissue. It can be caused by infections, autoimmune diseases, or medications and can lead to impaired kidney function.

Obstructive Nephropathy: Conditions such as kidney stones, tumors, or enlarged prostate glands can obstruct the flow of urine from the kidneys, leading to kidney damage over time.

Symptoms of Stage 4 Renal Disease

Stage 4 renal disease, or Stage 4 chronic kidney disease (CKD), is characterized by significantly reduced kidney function, typically with a glomerular filtration rate (GFR) of 15-29 mL/min/1.73m².

As kidney function declines, various symptoms may manifest, indicating the need for medical attention. Some common symptoms of Stage 4 renal disease include:

Fatigue and Weakness: Seniors with Stage 4 renal disease often experience persistent fatigue and weakness due to the buildup of waste products and electrolyte imbalances in the body.

Fluid Retention: Edema, or swelling, commonly occurs in the legs, ankles, and feet as the kidneys struggle to regulate fluid balance, leading to fluid retention.

Decreased Urination: Seniors may notice a decrease in urine output or changes in urinary frequency as kidney function declines.

Shortness of Breath: Fluid buildup in the lungs, known as pulmonary edema, can cause difficulty breathing or shortness of breath, especially during physical activity or when lying down.

High Blood Pressure: Uncontrolled hypertension is a common complication of Stage 4 renal disease, contributing to further kidney damage and cardiovascular issues.

Nausea and Vomiting: Seniors may experience nausea, vomiting, or loss of appetite due to the accumulation of waste products in the blood.

Itching and Skin Rash: Accumulation of waste products and electrolyte imbalances can cause itching, dry skin, or skin rashes.

Muscle Cramps and Restless Legs: Electrolyte imbalances and mineral deficiencies can lead to muscle cramps, twitching, or restless legs syndrome.

Risk Factor of Stage 4 Renal Disease

Stage 4 renal disease, or Stage 4 chronic kidney disease (CKD), can develop due to a combination of genetic, environmental, and lifestyle factors.

Several risk factors increase the likelihood of developing Stage 4 renal disease:

Diabetes Mellitus: Diabetes is the leading cause of CKD worldwide.

Prolonged high blood sugar levels can damage the small blood vessels in the kidneys, leading to diabetic nephropathy and CKD progression.

Hypertension (High Blood Pressure): Uncontrolled hypertension is a significant risk factor for CKD. Chronic high blood pressure can damage the blood vessels in the kidneys, impairing their ability to filter waste products from the blood effectively.

Family History: A family history of kidney disease or genetic disorders such as polycystic kidney disease (PKD) increases the risk of developing CKD.

Age: The risk of CKD increases with age, with older adults being more susceptible to kidney damage and decline in kidney function.

Obesity: Excess weight and obesity are associated with an increased risk of CKD, hypertension, and diabetes, all of which can contribute to kidney damage.

Smoking: Smoking tobacco increases the risk of CKD and accelerates kidney function decline, particularly in individuals with diabetes or hypertension.

Cardiovascular Disease: Conditions like heart disease, atherosclerosis, and peripheral vascular disease can impair kidney function and increase the risk of CKD.

CHAPTER TWO

Stage 4 Renal Diet Breakfast Recipes

1. Veggie Omelette

Ingredients:

* 2 eggs
* 1/4 cup diced bell peppers
* 1/4 cup diced onions
* 1/4 cup diced tomatoes
* Salt and pepper to taste
* 1 teaspoon olive oil

Instructions:

* In a bowl, beat the eggs with salt and pepper.
* Heat olive oil in a non-stick pan over medium heat.
* Add bell peppers, onions, and tomatoes to the pan and sauté until tender.
* Pour the beaten eggs into the pan, swirling to evenly distribute the vegetables.
* Cook until the edges are set, then flip the omelette and cook until fully cooked through.

* Serve hot with a side of whole grain toast or a slice of melon.

Health Benefits:

* This protein-rich breakfast provides essential amino acids for muscle health while incorporating colorful vegetables for added vitamins, minerals, and antioxidants.

Preparation Time: 15 minutes.

2. Greek Yogurt Parfait

Ingredients:

* 1/2 cup low-fat Greek yogurt
* 1/4 cup fresh berries (such as strawberries, blueberries, or raspberries)
* 1 tablespoon chopped nuts (such as almonds or walnuts)
* 1 teaspoon honey (optional)

Instructions:

* In a serving glass or bowl, layer Greek yogurt, fresh berries, and chopped nuts.

* Drizzle with honey if desired.
* Repeat the layers if using a larger container.
* Serve chilled.

Health Benefits:

* Greek yogurt provides high-quality protein with less potassium than traditional yogurt, while berries offer fiber and antioxidants.
* Nuts add healthy fats and crunch.

Preparation Time: 5 minutes.

3. Quinoa Breakfast Bowl

Ingredients:

* 1/2 cup cooked quinoa
* 1/4 cup sliced bananas
* 1 tablespoon chopped almonds
* 1 tablespoon raisins
* Cinnamon to taste
* 1/4 cup low-fat milk or almond milk (optional)

Instructions:

* In a bowl, combine cooked quinoa, sliced bananas, chopped almonds, and raisins.
* Sprinkle with cinnamon to taste.
* Add low-fat milk or almond milk if desired for creaminess.
* Stir gently to combine.
* Serve warm or chilled.

Health Benefits:

* Quinoa is a complete protein source and a good source of fiber, while bananas provide potassium and almonds offer healthy fats and vitamin E.

Preparation Time: 10 minutes.

4. Egg Muffin Cups

Ingredients:

* 4 eggs
* 1/4 cup diced bell peppers
* 1/4 cup diced onions
* 1/4 cup chopped spinach

* Salt and pepper to taste
* Cooking spray or olive oil

Instructions:

* Preheat the oven to 350°F (175°C) and lightly grease a muffin tin with cooking spray or olive oil.
* In a bowl, beat the eggs with salt and pepper.
* Stir in diced bell peppers, onions, and chopped spinach.
* Pour the egg mixture evenly into the muffin cups, filling each about 3/4 full.
* Bake in the preheated oven for 15-20 minutes or until the egg muffins are set and lightly golden on top.
* Allow to cool slightly before removing from the muffin tin.
* Serve warm or store in the refrigerator for later use.

Health Benefits:

* These egg muffin cups provide protein, vitamins, and minerals from eggs and vegetables in a convenient grab-and-go format.

Preparation Time: 25 minutes.

5. Overnight Oats

Ingredients:

* 1/2 cup old-fashioned rolled oats
* 1/2 cup low-fat milk or almond milk
* 1/4 cup Greek yogurt
* 1/4 cup sliced strawberries
* 1 tablespoon chia seeds
* 1 tablespoon honey or maple syrup (optional)

Instructions:

* In a jar or container, combine rolled oats, milk, Greek yogurt, sliced strawberries, chia seeds, and honey or maple syrup if using.
* Stir well to combine.
* Cover and refrigerate overnight or for at least 4 hours.
* In the morning, give the oats a good stir and add more milk if desired for a creamier consistency.
* Top with additional sliced strawberries before serving if desired.

Health Benefits:

* Overnight oats offer a nutritious and customizable breakfast option rich in fiber, protein, and omega-3 fatty acids from oats, Greek yogurt, and chia seeds.

Preparation Time: 5 minutes (plus overnight soaking).

6. Avocado Toast

Ingredients:

* 1 slice whole grain bread
* 1/4 ripe avocado
* 1 teaspoon lemon juice
* Pinch of salt and black pepper
* Optional toppings: sliced tomatoes, cucumber, radishes, or a sprinkle of hemp seeds

Instructions:

* Toast the slice of whole grain bread until golden brown.
* In a small bowl, mash the ripe avocado with lemon juice, salt, and black pepper until smooth.
* Spread the mashed avocado evenly onto the toasted bread.

* Top with sliced tomatoes, cucumber, radishes, or hemp seeds if desired.
* Serve immediately.

Health Benefits:

* Avocado toast provides healthy fats, fiber, and essential vitamins and minerals, making it a satisfying and nutritious breakfast choice.

Preparation Time: 5 minutes.

7. Berry Smoothie

Ingredients:

* 1/2 cup mixed berries (such as strawberries, blueberries, raspberries)
* 1/2 banana, sliced
* 1/2 cup low-fat Greek yogurt
* 1/2 cup low-fat milk or almond milk
* 1 tablespoon chia seeds (optional)
* 1 teaspoon honey or maple syrup (optional)

Instructions:

* In a blender, combine mixed berries, sliced banana, Greek yogurt, milk, chia seeds, and honey or maple syrup if using.
* Blend until smooth and creamy.
* If the smoothie is too thick, add more milk to reach the desired consistency.
* Pour into a glass and serve immediately.

Health Benefits:

* This berry smoothie is rich in antioxidants, fiber, and protein, providing a refreshing and nutritious breakfast option.

Preparation Time: 5 minutes.

8. Spinach and Feta Frittata

Ingredients:

* 4 eggs
* 1/4 cup chopped spinach
* 2 tablespoons crumbled feta cheese
* Salt and pepper to taste

* 1 teaspoon olive oil

Instructions:

* Preheat the oven to 350°F (175°C).
* In a bowl, beat the eggs with salt and pepper.
* Stir in chopped spinach and crumbled feta cheese.
* Heat olive oil in an oven-safe skillet over medium heat.
* Pour the egg mixture into the skillet and cook for 2-3 minutes until the edges begin to set.
* Transfer the skillet to the preheated oven and bake for 10-12 minutes or until the frittata is set and lightly golden on top.
* Remove from the oven and let cool slightly before slicing.
* Serve warm or at room temperature.

Health Benefits:

* This spinach and feta frittata is packed with protein, vitamins, and minerals from eggs and spinach, making it a nutritious breakfast option.

Preparation Time: 20 minutes.

9. Cottage Cheese and Fruit Bowl

Ingredients:

* 1/2 cup low-fat cottage cheese
* 1/2 cup diced mixed fruits (such as pineapple, melon, berries)
* 1 tablespoon chopped nuts (such as almonds or walnuts)
* 1 teaspoon honey or maple syrup (optional)

Instructions:

* In a serving bowl, layer low-fat cottage cheese, diced mixed fruits, and chopped nuts.
* Drizzle with honey or maple syrup if desired.
* Serve chilled.

Health Benefits:

* This cottage cheese and fruit bowl is rich in protein, vitamins, minerals, and antioxidants, offering a satisfying and nutritious breakfast option.

Preparation Time: 5 minutes.

10. Banana Nut Porridge

Ingredients:

* 1/2 cup old-fashioned rolled oats
* 1 cup water or low-fat milk
* 1/2 ripe banana, mashed
* 1 tablespoon chopped nuts (such as walnuts or almonds)
* Pinch of cinnamon
* 1 teaspoon honey or maple syrup (optional)

Instructions:

* In a saucepan, bring water or low-fat milk to a boil.
* Stir in old-fashioned rolled oats and reduce heat to low.
* Cook for 3-5 minutes, stirring occasionally, until the oats are creamy and tender.
* Stir in mashed banana, chopped nuts, cinnamon, and honey or maple syrup if desired.
* Cook for an additional 1-2 minutes until heated through.
* Remove from heat and let cool slightly before serving.

* Garnish with additional sliced banana or nuts if desired.

Health Benefits:

* This banana nut porridge is rich in fiber, protein, healthy fats, and essential vitamins and minerals, providing a comforting and nutritious breakfast option.

Preparation Time: 10 minutes.

Stage 4 Renal Diet Lunch Recipes

1. Grilled Chicken Salad

Ingredients:

* 3 oz grilled chicken breast, sliced
* 2 cups mixed salad greens
* 1/4 cup cherry tomatoes, halved
* 1/4 cucumber, sliced
* 1/4 avocado, diced
* 1 tablespoon sliced almonds
* Balsamic vinaigrette dressing (low-sodium)

Instructions:

* Arrange mixed salad greens on a plate.
* Top with grilled chicken breast slices, cherry tomatoes, cucumber slices, and diced avocado.
* Sprinkle with sliced almonds.
* Drizzle with balsamic vinaigrette dressing.
* Serve immediately.

Health Benefits:

* This grilled chicken salad is rich in lean protein, fiber, vitamins, minerals, and healthy fats, providing a nutritious and satisfying lunch option.

Preparation Time: 15 minutes.

2. Turkey and Veggie Wrap

Ingredients:

* 2 slices whole grain tortilla
* 3 oz deli turkey breast slices
* 1/4 cup shredded lettuce
* 1/4 cup sliced bell peppers
* 1/4 cup shredded carrots

* 1 tablespoon hummus (low-sodium)

Instructions:

* Lay out whole grain tortillas on a clean surface.
* Spread hummus evenly on each tortilla.
* Layer deli turkey breast slices, shredded lettuce, sliced bell peppers, and shredded carrots on top of the hummus.
* Roll up the tortillas tightly, enclosing the filling.
* Slice each wrap in half diagonally.
* Serve immediately or wrap in foil for later.

Health Benefits:

* This turkey and veggie wrap is packed with lean protein, fiber, vitamins, minerals, and antioxidants, offering a nutritious and portable lunch option.

Preparation Time: 10 minutes.

3. Tuna Salad Stuffed Tomato

Ingredients:

* 1 large tomato
* 1/2 cup canned tuna, drained

* 1 tablespoon diced celery
* 1 tablespoon diced red onion
* 1 tablespoon chopped parsley
* 1 tablespoon mayonnaise (low-fat)

Instructions:

* Cut the top off the tomato and scoop out the seeds and pulp to create a hollow cavity.
* In a bowl, mix canned tuna, diced celery, diced red onion, chopped parsley, and mayonnaise until well combined.
* Spoon the tuna salad mixture into the hollowed-out tomato.
* Serve immediately or chill in the refrigerator until ready to eat.

Health Benefits:

* This tuna salad stuffed tomato is a low-calorie, protein-rich option packed with essential nutrients, vitamins, and minerals, offering a light and refreshing lunch choice.

Preparation Time: 10 minutes.

4. Quinoa Salad with Chickpeas

Ingredients:

* 1/2 cup cooked quinoa
* 1/4 cup canned chickpeas, drained and rinsed
* 1/4 cup diced cucumber
* 1/4 cup diced bell peppers
* 2 tablespoons chopped fresh parsley
* 1 tablespoon olive oil
* 1 tablespoon lemon juice
* Salt and pepper to taste

Instructions:

* In a bowl, combine cooked quinoa, chickpeas, diced cucumber, diced bell peppers, and chopped fresh parsley.
* Drizzle with olive oil and lemon juice.
* Season with salt and pepper to taste.
* Toss gently until well combined.
* Serve chilled or at room temperature.

Health Benefits:

* This quinoa salad with chickpeas is rich in plant-based protein, fiber, vitamins, minerals, and healthy fats, providing a nutritious and filling lunch option.

Preparation Time: 15 minutes.

5. Vegetable Stir-Fry

Ingredients:

* 1/2 cup mixed vegetables (such as bell peppers, broccoli, carrots, snap peas)
* 3 oz tofu, diced
* 1 tablespoon low-sodium soy sauce
* 1 teaspoon sesame oil
* 1 teaspoon minced garlic
* Cooked brown rice (optional)

Instructions:

* Heat sesame oil in a skillet or wok over medium-high heat.
* Add minced garlic and diced tofu to the skillet and stir-fry until tofu is lightly browned.

* Add mixed vegetables to the skillet and continue to stir-fry until vegetables are tender-crisp.
* Drizzle with low-sodium soy sauce and toss until evenly coated.
* Serve vegetable stir-fry hot over cooked brown rice if desired.

Health Benefits:

* This vegetable stir-fry is loaded with fiber, vitamins, minerals, and plant-based protein, providing a nutritious and flavorful lunch option.

Preparation Time: 15 minutes.

6. Lentil Soup

Ingredients:

* 1/2 cup dried lentils
* 2 cups low-sodium vegetable broth
* 1/4 cup diced onions
* 1/4 cup diced carrots
* 1/4 cup diced celery
* 1 teaspoon minced garlic
* 1 bay leaf

* Salt and pepper to taste

* Chopped fresh parsley for garnish

Instructions:

* Rinse dried lentils under cold water and drain well.

* In a pot, combine lentils, low-sodium vegetable broth, diced onions, diced carrots, diced celery, minced garlic, and bay leaf.

* Bring to a boil over medium-high heat, then reduce heat to low and simmer for 20-25 minutes or until lentils are tender.

* Season with salt and pepper to taste.

* Remove bay leaf before serving.

* Garnish with chopped fresh parsley.

* Serve hot.

Health Benefits:

* This lentil soup is a nutritious and hearty option rich in fiber, protein, vitamins, minerals, and antioxidants, offering a comforting and satisfying lunch choice.

Preparation Time: 30 minutes.

7. Salmon and Quinoa Bowl

Ingredients:

* 3 oz baked or grilled salmon fillet
* 1/2 cup cooked quinoa
* 1/4 cup steamed broccoli florets
* 1/4 cup sliced cherry tomatoes
* 1 tablespoon chopped fresh dill
* Lemon wedges for serving

Instructions:

* In a bowl, combine cooked quinoa, steamed broccoli florets, sliced cherry tomatoes, and chopped fresh dill.
* Place baked or grilled salmon fillet on top of the quinoa mixture.
* Serve with lemon wedges on the side.
* Serve immediately.

Health Benefits:

* This salmon and quinoa bowl is a nutrient-rich meal loaded with omega-3 fatty acids, protein, fiber,

vitamins, minerals, and antioxidants, offering a delicious and satisfying lunch option.

Preparation Time: 20 minutes.

8. Egg Salad Lettuce Wraps

Ingredients:

* 2 hard-boiled eggs, chopped
* 2 tablespoons Greek yogurt
* 1 tablespoon chopped celery
* 1 tablespoon chopped red onion
* Salt and pepper to taste
* 4 large lettuce leaves (such as romaine or butter lettuce)

Instructions:

* In a bowl, combine chopped hard-boiled eggs, Greek yogurt, chopped celery, and chopped red onion.
* Season with salt and pepper to taste.
* Spoon the egg salad mixture onto large lettuce leaves.
* Roll up the lettuce leaves to form wraps.
* Serve immediately.

Health Benefits:

*   These egg salad lettuce wraps are low in calories and carbohydrates while providing protein, vitamins, minerals, and healthy fats, offering a light and refreshing lunch option.

Preparation Time: 15 minutes.

9. Chicken and Vegetable Stir-Fry

Ingredients:

*   3 oz cooked chicken breast, sliced
*   1/2 cup mixed vegetables (such as bell peppers, snap peas, carrots)
*   1 tablespoon low-sodium soy sauce
*   1 teaspoon sesame oil
*   1 teaspoon minced ginger
*   1 teaspoon minced garlic
*   Cooked brown rice (optional)

Instructions:

*   Heat sesame oil in a skillet or wok over medium-high heat.

* Add minced ginger and minced garlic to the skillet and stir-fry until fragrant.
* Add sliced chicken breast and mixed vegetables to the skillet and stir-fry until chicken is heated through and vegetables are tender-crisp.
* Drizzle with low-sodium soy sauce and toss until evenly coated.
* Serve chicken and vegetable stir-fry hot over cooked brown rice if desired.

Health Benefits:

* This chicken and vegetable stir-fry is a nutritious and flavorful option rich in lean protein, fiber, vitamins, minerals, and antioxidants, providing a satisfying and balanced lunch choice.

Preparation Time: 20 minutes.

10. Caprese Salad

Ingredients:

* 1 large tomato, sliced
* 1/4 cup fresh mozzarella cheese, sliced
* 1/4 cup fresh basil leaves

* 1 tablespoon balsamic glaze (low-sodium)
* Salt and pepper to taste

Instructions:

* Arrange sliced tomatoes, fresh mozzarella cheese, and fresh basil leaves on a serving plate.
* Drizzle with balsamic glaze.
* Season with salt and pepper to taste.
* Serve immediately.

Health Benefits:

* This Caprese salad is a light and refreshing option packed with vitamins, minerals, and antioxidants from fresh tomatoes, mozzarella cheese, and basil, offering a flavorful and satisfying lunch choice.

Preparation Time: 10 minutes.

Stage 4 Renal Diet Dinner Recipes

1. Grilled Lemon Herb Salmon

Ingredients:

* 1 salmon fillet (4-6 ounces)
* 1 tablespoon lemon juice

* 1 teaspoon olive oil
* 1 teaspoon chopped fresh herbs (such as parsley, dill, or thyme)
* Salt and pepper to taste

Instructions:

* Preheat the grill to medium-high heat.
* In a small bowl, mix together lemon juice, olive oil, chopped herbs, salt, and pepper.
* Brush the mixture onto the salmon fillet.
* Place the salmon fillet on the preheated grill and cook for 4-5 minutes per side, or until the salmon is cooked through and flakes easily with a fork.
* Serve hot with steamed vegetables and quinoa or brown rice.

Health Benefits:

* Salmon is rich in omega-3 fatty acids, protein, and vitamins D and B12, while fresh herbs add flavor without excess sodium.

Preparation Time: 15 minutes.

2. Vegetable Stir-Fry

Ingredients:

* 1 cup mixed vegetables (such as bell peppers, broccoli, carrots, snap peas)
* 1 tablespoon olive oil
* 2 cloves garlic, minced
* 1 teaspoon grated ginger
* 2 tablespoons low-sodium soy sauce
* 1 teaspoon sesame oil
* Cooked brown rice or quinoa for serving

Instructions:

* Heat olive oil in a large skillet or wok over medium-high heat.
* Add minced garlic and grated ginger to the skillet and cook for 1-2 minutes, until fragrant.
* Add mixed vegetables to the skillet and stir-fry for 5-6 minutes, until tender-crisp.
* Stir in low-sodium soy sauce and sesame oil, tossing to coat the vegetables evenly.
* Cook for an additional 1-2 minutes, then remove from heat.

* Serve hot over cooked brown rice or quinoa.

Health Benefits:

* This vegetable stir-fry is packed with fiber, vitamins, and minerals from a variety of colorful vegetables, providing a nutritious and satisfying meal.

Preparation Time: 20 minutes.

3. Baked Chicken Breast

Ingredients:

* 1 boneless, skinless chicken breast
* 1 tablespoon olive oil
* 1 teaspoon garlic powder
* 1 teaspoon paprika
* 1/2 teaspoon dried thyme
* Salt and pepper to taste

Instructions:

* Preheat the oven to 375°F (190°C).
* Place the chicken breast on a baking sheet lined with parchment paper.

* Drizzle olive oil over the chicken breast and rub to coat evenly.

* In a small bowl, mix together garlic powder, paprika, dried thyme, salt, and pepper.

* Sprinkle the seasoning mixture over the chicken breast, rubbing to coat both sides.

* Bake in the preheated oven for 20-25 minutes, or until the chicken is cooked through and reaches an internal temperature of 165°F (75°C).

* Let the chicken rest for a few minutes before slicing.

* Serve hot with steamed vegetables and a side salad.

Health Benefits:

* Baked chicken breast is a lean protein source, while herbs and spices add flavor without excess sodium or fat.

Preparation Time: 30 minutes.

4. Lentil Vegetable Soup

Ingredients:

* 1/2 cup dried green lentils
* 4 cups low-sodium vegetable broth

* 1 cup mixed vegetables (such as carrots, celery, onions)
* 2 cloves garlic, minced
* 1 teaspoon olive oil
* 1 teaspoon dried thyme
* Salt and pepper to taste
* Fresh parsley for garnish (optional)

Instructions:

* Rinse the dried green lentils under cold water and drain.
* Heat olive oil in a large pot over medium heat.
* Add minced garlic to the pot and cook for 1-2 minutes, until fragrant.
* Add mixed vegetables to the pot and sauté for 5-6 minutes, until tender.
* Stir in dried green lentils, vegetable broth, dried thyme, salt, and pepper.
* Bring the soup to a boil, then reduce heat to low and simmer for 25-30 minutes, or until the lentils are tender.
* Adjust seasoning to taste.

* Serve hot, garnished with fresh parsley if desired.

Health Benefits:

* Lentil vegetable soup is rich in fiber, protein, vitamins, and minerals, providing a hearty and nutritious meal.

Preparation Time: 40 minutes.

5. Turkey and Vegetable Skewers

Ingredients:

* 4 ounces turkey breast, cut into cubes
* 1/2 cup mixed vegetables (such as bell peppers, zucchini, mushrooms)
* 1 tablespoon olive oil
* 1 teaspoon dried oregano
* Salt and pepper to taste
* Lemon wedges for serving

Instructions:

* Preheat the grill or grill pan to medium-high heat.
* Thread turkey cubes and mixed vegetables onto skewers, alternating as desired.

* Brush skewers with olive oil and sprinkle with dried oregano, salt, and pepper.

* Grill skewers for 8-10 minutes, turning occasionally, until the turkey is cooked through and vegetables are tender.

* Serve hot with lemon wedges for squeezing over the skewers.

Health Benefits:

* Turkey and vegetable skewers provide lean protein, fiber, vitamins, and minerals, offering a flavorful and nutritious dinner option.

Preparation Time: 20 minutes.

6. Eggplant Parmesan

Ingredients:

* 1 small eggplant, sliced into rounds
* 1 egg, beaten
* 1/2 cup whole wheat breadcrumbs
* 1/4 cup grated Parmesan cheese
* 1 cup low-sodium marinara sauce
* 1/2 cup shredded mozzarella cheese

* 1 teaspoon dried Italian seasoning

* Olive oil cooking spray

Instructions:

* Preheat the oven to 375°F (190°C) and line a baking sheet with parchment paper.

* Dip eggplant slices into beaten egg, then coat with a mixture of whole wheat breadcrumbs and grated Parmesan cheese.

* Place coated eggplant slices on the prepared baking sheet and spray lightly with olive oil cooking spray.

* Bake in the preheated oven for 20-25 minutes, or until the eggplant is tender and the coating is golden brown.

* Remove from the oven and top each eggplant slice with a spoonful of marinara sauce and a sprinkle of shredded mozzarella cheese.

* Return to the oven and bake for an additional 5-7 minutes, or until the cheese is melted and bubbly.

* Sprinkle with dried Italian seasoning before serving.

Health Benefits:

* Eggplant Parmesan is a lighter version of the classic Italian dish, providing fiber, vitamins, and minerals from eggplant and whole wheat breadcrumbs, with less saturated fat and sodium.

Preparation Time: 35 minutes.

7. Lemon Garlic Shrimp Pasta

Ingredients:

* 4 ounces whole wheat spaghetti or linguine
* 8 ounces shrimp, peeled and deveined
* 2 cloves garlic, minced
* 1 tablespoon olive oil
* 1 tablespoon lemon juice
* Zest of 1 lemon
* Salt and pepper to taste
* Fresh parsley for garnish (optional)

Instructions:

* Cook whole wheat spaghetti or linguine according to package instructions until al dente.

* Meanwhile, heat olive oil in a large skillet over medium heat.
* Add minced garlic to the skillet and cook for 1-2 minutes, until fragrant.
* Add shrimp to the skillet and cook for 2-3 minutes on each side, until pink and opaque.
* Stir in lemon juice and zest, tossing to coat the shrimp evenly.
* Season with salt and pepper to taste.
* Drain cooked pasta and add to the skillet, tossing to combine with the shrimp and lemon garlic sauce.
* Serve hot, garnished with fresh parsley if desired.

Health Benefits:

* Lemon garlic shrimp pasta provides lean protein, whole grains, and citrus flavor, making it a flavorful and satisfying dinner option.

Preparation Time: 20 minutes.

8. Baked Cod with Tomatoes and Olives

Ingredients:

* 1 cod fillet (4-6 ounces)

* 1/2 cup cherry tomatoes, halved
* 1/4 cup sliced Kalamata olives
* 1 tablespoon olive oil
* 1 clove garlic, minced
* 1 teaspoon dried oregano
* Salt and pepper to taste
* Lemon wedges for serving

Instructions:

* Preheat the oven to 375°F (190°C) and line a baking sheet with parchment paper.
* Place the cod fillet on the prepared baking sheet.
* In a small bowl, mix together cherry tomatoes, sliced Kalamata olives, olive oil, minced garlic, dried oregano, salt, and pepper.
* Spoon the tomato and olive mixture over the cod fillet, covering evenly.
* Bake in the preheated oven for 12-15 minutes, or until the cod is cooked through and flakes easily with a fork.
* Serve hot with lemon wedges for squeezing over the fish.

Health Benefits:

* Baked cod with tomatoes and olives offers lean protein, heart-healthy fats, and antioxidants from fish and vegetables, making it a nutritious and flavorful dinner option.

Preparation Time: 20 minutes.

9. Spinach and Mushroom Quiche

Ingredients:

* 1 whole wheat pie crust
* 4 eggs
* 1 cup low-fat milk or almond milk
* 1 cup chopped spinach
* 1/2 cup sliced mushrooms
* 1/4 cup diced onions
* 1/2 cup shredded mozzarella cheese
* Salt and pepper to taste
* Olive oil cooking spray

Instructions:

* Preheat the oven to 375°F (190°C).

* Place the whole wheat pie crust in a pie dish and set aside.
* In a skillet, sauté chopped spinach, sliced mushrooms, and diced onions over medium heat until softened.
* In a bowl, whisk together eggs, low-fat milk, shredded mozzarella cheese, salt, and pepper.
* Stir in sautéed spinach, mushrooms, and onions.
* Pour the egg mixture into the prepared pie crust.
* Bake in the preheated oven for 30-35 minutes, or until the quiche is set and golden brown on top.
* Let cool slightly before slicing and serving.

Health Benefits:

* Spinach and mushroom quiche provides protein, fiber, vitamins, and minerals from eggs, vegetables, and whole grains, making it a nutritious and satisfying dinner option.

Preparation Time: 45 minutes.

10. Chicken and Vegetable Curry

Ingredients:

* 4 ounces chicken breast, cut into cubes
* 1 cup mixed vegetables (such as bell peppers, carrots, peas)
* 1/2 cup light coconut milk
* 1 tablespoon curry powder
* 1 clove garlic, minced
* 1 teaspoon grated ginger
* 1 tablespoon olive oil
* Cooked brown rice for serving

Instructions:

* Heat olive oil in a skillet over medium heat.
* Add minced garlic and grated ginger to the skillet and cook for 1-2 minutes, until fragrant.
* Add chicken cubes to the skillet and cook for 5-6 minutes, until browned on all sides.
* Stir in mixed vegetables and curry powder, tossing to coat evenly.
* Add light coconut milk to the skillet and bring to a simmer.

* Cover and cook for 10-12 minutes, or until the chicken is cooked through and vegetables are tender.
* Serve hot over cooked brown rice.

Health Benefits:

* Chicken and vegetable curry is rich in protein, fiber, vitamins, and minerals from chicken, vegetables, and spices, offering a flavorful and nutritious dinner option.

Preparation Time: 30 minutes.

Stage 4 Renal Diet Snacks Recipes

1. Greek Yogurt with Berries

Ingredients:

* 1/2 cup low-fat Greek yogurt
* 1/4 cup mixed berries (such as strawberries, blueberries, raspberries)
* 1 tablespoon chopped almonds or walnuts
* 1 teaspoon honey or maple syrup (optional)

Instructions: In a bowl, layer low-fat Greek yogurt with mixed berries.

* Sprinkle chopped almonds or walnuts on top.
* Drizzle with honey or maple syrup if desired.
* Serve immediately.

Health Benefits:

* This snack provides protein, fiber, and antioxidants from Greek yogurt, berries, and nuts, offering a satisfying and nutritious option.

Preparation Time: 5 minutes.

2. Rice Cake with Peanut Butter and Banana

Ingredients:

* 1 rice cake
* 1 tablespoon peanut butter (unsalted)
* 1/2 banana, sliced

Instructions:

* Spread peanut butter evenly on top of the rice cake.
* Arrange sliced banana on top of the peanut butter.
* Serve immediately.

Health Benefits:

* This snack provides a combination of protein, healthy fats, and carbohydrates, making it a quick and energizing option.

Preparation Time: 2 minutes.

3. Cottage Cheese with Pineapple

Ingredients:

* 1/2 cup low-fat cottage cheese
* 1/4 cup diced pineapple (fresh or canned in juice, drained)

Instructions:

* In a bowl, combine low-fat cottage cheese with diced pineapple.
* Mix well.
* Serve chilled.

Health Benefits: This snack is rich in protein, calcium, and vitamin C, offering a refreshing and nutritious option.

Preparation Time: 3 minutes.

4. Veggie Sticks with Hummus

Ingredients:

* 1/2 cup mixed vegetable sticks (such as carrots, celery, bell peppers)
* 2 tablespoons hummus (low-sodium)

Instructions:

* Arrange mixed vegetable sticks on a plate.
* Serve with hummus for dipping.
* Enjoy!

Health Benefits:

* This snack is rich in fiber, vitamins, and minerals from vegetables, while hummus provides protein and healthy fats.

Preparation Time: 5 minutes.

5. Hard-Boiled Egg

Ingredients:

* 1 hard-boiled egg

Instructions: Place egg in a saucepan and cover with water.

* Bring water to a boil, then reduce heat and simmer for 10 minutes.
* Remove egg from water and let cool before peeling.
* Enjoy as is or with a sprinkle of salt and pepper if desired.

Health Benefits:

* Hard-boiled eggs are an excellent source of protein and essential nutrients, making them a convenient and nutritious snack option.

Preparation Time: 15 minutes.

6. Trail Mix

Ingredients:

* 1/4 cup mixed nuts (such as almonds, walnuts, cashews)
* 2 tablespoons dried fruit (such as raisins, cranberries)
* 1 tablespoon pumpkin seeds

Instructions:

* In a bowl, combine mixed nuts, dried fruit, and pumpkin seeds.

* Mix well.
* Portion into individual servings or store in an airtight container for later use.
* Enjoy as a quick and portable snack.

Health Benefits:

* Trail mix provides a mix of protein, healthy fats, and carbohydrates, offering a satisfying and energizing option.

Preparation Time: 2 minutes.

7. Apple Slices with Almond Butter

Ingredients:

* 1 small apple, sliced
* 1 tablespoon almond butter (unsalted)

Instructions:

* Spread almond butter on apple slices.
* Serve immediately.

Health Benefits: This snack offers a combination of fiber, vitamins, minerals, and healthy fats, providing a delicious and nutritious option.

Preparation Time: 3 minutes.

8. Cucumber and Tomato Salad

Ingredients:

* 1 small cucumber, sliced
* 1 small tomato, diced
* 1 tablespoon chopped fresh parsley
* 1 teaspoon olive oil
* 1 teaspoon lemon juice
* Salt and pepper to taste

Instructions:

* In a bowl, combine cucumber slices, diced tomato, and chopped parsley.
* Drizzle with olive oil and lemon juice.
* Season with salt and pepper to taste.
* Toss gently to combine.
* Serve immediately.

Health Benefits: This refreshing salad provides hydration, fiber, vitamins, and antioxidants from cucumber, tomato, and parsley.

Preparation Time: 5 minutes.

9. Tuna Salad on Crackers

Ingredients:

* 1/4 cup canned tuna (packed in water, drained)
* 1 tablespoon plain Greek yogurt
* 1 teaspoon lemon juice
* Salt and pepper to taste
* 4 whole grain crackers

Instructions:

* In a bowl, mix canned tuna with Greek yogurt, lemon juice, salt, and pepper.
* Spread tuna salad evenly on whole grain crackers.
* Serve immediately.

Health Benefits:

* This snack is rich in protein, omega-3 fatty acids, and whole grains, providing a satisfying and nutritious option.

Preparation Time: 5 minutes.

10. Dark Chocolate Covered Almonds

Ingredients:

* 10 raw almonds
* 1 ounce dark chocolate (70% cocoa or higher)

Instructions:

* Melt dark chocolate in a microwave-safe bowl in 30-second intervals, stirring until smooth.
* Dip almonds into melted chocolate to coat.
* Place chocolate-covered almonds on a parchment-lined tray.
* Let cool until chocolate hardens.
* Enjoy as a sweet and satisfying snack.

Health Benefits:

* Dark chocolate provides antioxidants, while almonds offer protein, healthy fats, and fiber, making this snack a delicious and nutritious treat.

Preparation Time: 10 minutes.

CONCLUSION

This Stage 4 Renal Diet Cookbook for Seniors serves as a comprehensive guide, offering a diverse array of delicious and nutritious recipes tailored specifically for individuals managing advanced kidney disease.

Through careful consideration of nutrient restrictions and dietary guidelines, each recipe is thoughtfully crafted to support kidney health while providing enjoyable meal options for seniors.

By incorporating a variety of wholesome ingredients and creative cooking techniques, this cookbook aims to make adhering to the renal diet more manageable and enjoyable for seniors.

From satisfying breakfast options to convenient snacks and hearty main dishes, there's something for every mealtime and occasion.

Moreover, beyond just providing recipes, this cookbook empowers seniors with valuable knowledge about the principles of the Stage 4 renal diet, understanding the importance of nutrient control, and practical tips for meal planning and preparation.

It emphasizes the significance of collaboration with healthcare professionals and encourages individuals to take an active role in managing their health through informed dietary choices.

Ultimately, this cookbook is not just about nourishing the body; it's about nurturing well-being and enhancing quality of life.

Whether you're seeking a comforting bowl of oatmeal, a flavorful vegetable stir-fry, or a refreshing fruit smoothie, these recipes are designed to inspire and support seniors on their journey to better kidney health.

With each bite, may you find nourishment, satisfaction, and the joy of culinary creativity.